"I think all doctors get upset when a patient loses an eye. We see it as failure to save sight. Thank you for allowing me to read your mini- memoir. This will be helpful for many people."

~**Anonymous**

"Sometimes I run into one of my patients in the 'real world,' away from the office mirrors, bright lights and the constant critiquing of details. When I have a conversation with the patient or see them from a distance socializing or shopping, I may notice my work, but no one else around is looking at it. In fact, most of us have seen someone, or met someone, who wears an ocular prosthesis without ever noticing.

The combination of modern surgical techniques, technology, and artistry has made the typical wearer of an ocular prosthesis practically invisible. Even so, the loss of an eye is usually tragic and can be quite devastating. Often, by the time a patient reaches my office, the grief has run its course and acceptance and excitement take its place.

In her writing, Cynthia De Boer brings the reader into her world where emotions of tragedy, insecurity, and eventual acceptance are displayed and exposed for all to appreciate. The loss of an eye is indeed tragic; but like any adversity, I have more often seen the experience of my patients serve to make them stronger and wiser. Cynthia is a perfect example of one who has gained strength of character and a loving confident perspective from her adversities."

~**Eric M. Lindsey**, BCO Board Certified Ocularist, www.prosticartists.com, www.ericlindseyartist.com

"Cynthia De Boer's fascinating and inspiring chronicle truly captured the wonderful transition from the pain and fear of losing her eye to acceptance and even gratitude in adapting to a prosthetic eye. As someone who faced the challenge of complete hearing loss and consequent cochlear implant surgeries in both ears, followed by the extremely difficult adaptation to hearing electronic sounds, I feel Cynthia's unique insights will be educational and beneficial to those with similar life-altering physical challenges."

~**Bruce Woodbury**, Attorney, Boulder City Hospital Board of Trustees, St. Rose Hospital Community Board, former Clark County Nevada Commissioner

"When I was asked to read and comment on Cynthia De Boer's book, I did not know what to expect. What I found was a deeply personal and fascinating book about an unfamiliar subject.

Cynthia's honesty and detail will help anyone who is dealing with the issue of losing an eye, but it is more than just that. This book is a wonderful look at one person dealing with an issue few can comprehend, and making a success of it. Being a person who uses my eyes daily as a necessary part of my work, I cannot imagine what it would be like to lose one. But having this happen at seventeen, a vulnerable age at best for anyone, gives this story a punch I did not expect.

We all remember our teens, the era when we are trying to come to grips with who we are and what we were supposed to do. To lose an eye and have to learn to live with a prosthetic replacement would be unimaginable. Cynthia brings us inside a young woman's experience of such a loss, allowing the reader to feel what it meant to her. If you are looking for a book that will make you think about your own life, this one will do it. It may be short. But it is well worth reading. I am honored to be able to recommend it to anyone who wants to learn about loss and healing."

"Wow! I met Cyndi many years ago, and I was talking to her about health and diet and gave her some tips on how to eat healthy that were not in alignment with the popular diets of the time. I advised her to cut back on the carbs and never thought much about it again.

Sometime later, it must have been a few months; she noticed an improvement in her vision and told me about her prosthetic eye. This totally took me by surprise because I have vision in only one eye, and as a child had strabismus—"cross-eye" or "lazy eye"—as the doctors would call it. At six years of age they blamed it on me, and said that I was not doing all I could to use the lazy eye. It got to the point where I was "forced" to use the eye by patching the good eye. I don't remember how long that lasted, but I do remember feeling like I was living in a cloud. Everything looked cloudy white or grayish, and I was bumping into everything. After a while, they took my patch off, but I could no longer see with the "good" eye. Fortunately for me, over time, my vision in the good eye came back, though not perfect.

As I became an adult, I could tell by looking at people's eyes and the way they moved their heads if there was a lack of vision in one eye or not, but not with Cyndi. She had her movements down to perfection. Her attitude is amazing and *she* is absolutely amazing to have gone through the suffering with not a hint of complaining. She is truly brave and an example for all of us to follow.

I fixed my own strabismus by balancing the eye muscles. From childhood to this day I never liked glasses, so I don't wear them unless I need to read. Like Cyndi, I never speak about my lack of vision; in fact, I don't even like to think about it. I can count on one hand the number of people who know about it. So I can totally sympathize and identify with how she felt.

Even after reading Cyndi's story and knowing all the facts about her suffering, I never noticed telltale signs; I only saw a beautiful, radiant, light- hearted woman with a great sense of humor that warms everyone she comes in contact with."

~**Nick Prvulov**, Hypnotherapist,
Nutritional Consultant,
Bachelor of Science

"The author of this book, Cynthia De Boer, has written a wonderful story about herself and how she dealt with losing a God-given organ of her body, in her case an eye. She has personalized the book to show how perseverance and understanding can sustain one's sense of loss. The author has given back to everyone the knowledge and understanding to accept and press forward in a positive way to overcome any of life's adversities. This book should be read by every person who has, or has had, the misfortune of experiencing the loss of an organ such as the author has shared."

~**Ronald W. Keller**,
Professional Educator

"Wow! Cynthia addresses the impact on the patient, while allowing friends and family an opportunity to understand how to provide productive support. This book should help anticipate various events, both expected and unexpected, for all involved."

~**Marilyn Yeager**, Orthopedic Surgeon's
Office Manager

"As Cynthia mentioned in her book, our conversation about my phantom pain helped her understand this strange phenomenon; and now she is happily sharing this experience, and many others, with her readers. Cynthia's honest story gives encouragement and hope to everyone, particularly to those with a handicap as well as to their family members."

~**Richard W. Maynard**, Retired, Iowa
State/ Motor Fuel Tax Dept.

"Cynthia De Boer has written an unusual and encouraging story of her life plagued by severe blindness. Don't miss *Me, Myself and Eye* for a history of a successful life lived with courage and determination."

~**Sharon Peterson**, Former Teacher,
Flight Attendant and Polio Survivor

"*Me, Myself and Eye* takes you on a powerful soul- searching journey of a young girl's experiences enduring both losing her eye and wearing a prosthetic eye. She reaches deep inside herself to share not just the emotional side of her transition but the physical aspects of it as well. Cynthia shares all the knowledge she learned along the way in hopes it may help someone else that might have to go through the same thing. This book should be read by everyone because it empowers you to be selfless, brave, and to reach for the stars."

~**Penny Rea**, Artist,
www.ArtByPennyRea.com

"Cynthia De Boer is truly an inspiration to anyone who has gone through something so tragic in their lives. She took an extreme hardship and tragedy and turned it into a positive, and she didn't let any obstacle stand in her way! For her to experience such a loss, she was able to remain strong and accomplish so many great things in her life. Wow! What an amazing story and journey!

Me, Myself & Eye is a story *everyone* should read!"

~**Angela Christin Poulson**, Educator

"Through the story of *Me Myself & Eye*, we as readers follow Cyndi through what should be an impossible journey. With her unshakeable faith, we're witnesses to a strength and outpouring of compassion. Love and blessings surely follow her steps."

~**Cheryl Waites**,
Founder of Earth Angel Project

"I suspect many people will benefit from Cynthia Lee De Boer's short yet brave book. It's a perfect balance of practical and passionate."

~**Matthew O'Brien**, Author, *Beneath The Neon* and *My Week at the Blue Angel*, Adjunct Professor of English, UNLV.

"I love the heartfelt tone of Cyndi's book and know it will help many people throughout the world. This book pinpoints the hardships and emotions she had to endure and how she handled them. I'm sure it will give readers a very positive insight into how to deal with their struggles."

~Linda Korfman, Realtor

"An informational and inspiring guide about life with a prosthetic eye."

~Jenny Ballif, Freelance Writer

"In *Me, Myself & Eye*, Cynthia De Boer writes from the heart and shares some of her hardest and most trying times as a teenager. She is able to make you feel all of the emotions she went through with such a soft touch. This should be a helpful read to anyone going through the same life-changing event. Knowing Cyndi for over thirty years, it is an honor to be one of the first few people to read her inspiring story, and her strength will help many people."

~**Rick W. Stewart**

"*Me, Myself & Eye* is a tribute to the courage of a young girl dealing with adversity, fear, anxiety, and ridicule. Cynthia's perseverance and determination can be appreciated by anyone who has dealt with the pain of being different. She shares her story with the hope of helping others, particularly those facing the loss of an eye. Cynthia's example shows the power of love and support from family, friends, and dedicated professionals. Her recognition of the blessings realized clearly reflects that, while her eyesight is impaired, her spiritual sight has only sharpened."

~**Carol Cerrone Richards**, Author, *Take a Break Self-Meditate*

"Wow! What an inspiration! Cynthia L. De

Boer is a courageous woman for not only sharing her very personal experiences but for living through it with such determination. Her story will undoubtedly help countless others. A definite must-read. It will change your perspective, understanding, and level of compassion!"

~**Stephanie Tejada,** Founder,
www.StephaniesGourmet.com

"An absolute must-read for anyone facing eye surgery."

~**Jean Luttrell**, Author, *Riffey,
the Last Old Time Ranger*

"Honest, gripping, insightful. This well-written book, and the journey traveled by the author, is magnificently portrayed. The joy, the sadness, and acceptance culminate in the person Cynthia is today."

~**Hon-Vu Q. Duong**, MD, Clinical Instructor of Ophthalmology, Westfield Eye

Center; Senior Lecturer of Neuroscience, Anatomy & Physiology, Nevada State College

ME,
MYSELF
&EYE

ME,

MYSELF

&EYE

The Realities of Living With a Prosthetic Eye

Cynthia Lee De Boer

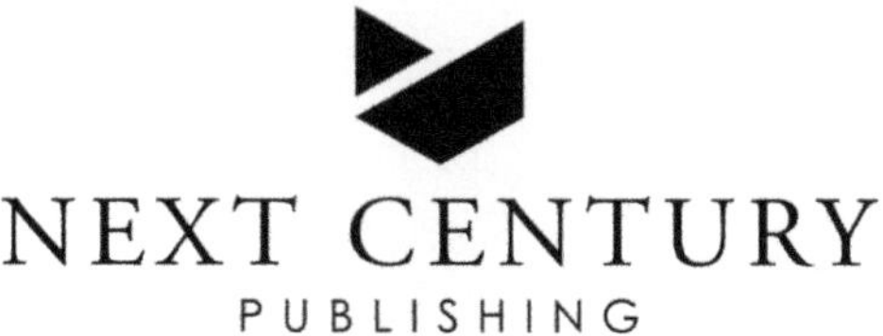

ME, MYSELF & EYE

The Realities of Living With a Prosthetic Eye

Published by Next Century Publishing Las Vegas, Nevada www.NextCenturyPublishing.com

ISBN: 978-1-68102-143-0

Printed in the United States of AmericaLibrary of Congress Control Number: 2016934569

DEDICATION

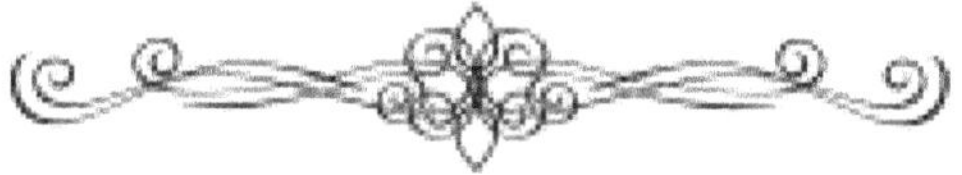

I am dedicating this informational mini- memoir to all my fellow one-eyed wonders. May your journeys be enlightening and your pleasures many. I hope we meet someday. I'll keep an "eye" out for you...

TABLE OF CONTENTS

ME, MYSELF & EYE

ACKNOWLEDGEMENTS

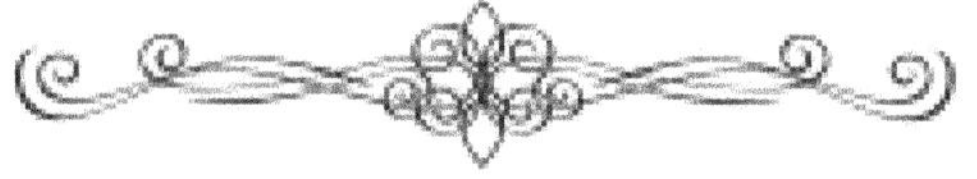

Reliving many difficult times as I brought my story to the page was quite painful. I often wondered if my readers would feel the importance I placed on this work. But I am compelled to write; I know there are countless people who have gone through, or are facing the same trial as I've dealt with. After all this is such a personal story and it's to be given to complete strangers. I kept coming back to the point in time when I found out I was going to lose my eye. It was terrifying and many frightening days followed. I felt if I could ease even one person's pain, mine would be of value. But the truth of the matter is this was an incredible struggle. There were days when I wanted to give it all up, and if not for the love and support of so many, this book would never be.

Sincere thanks to my loving husband Dann, my father Larry, my sister Penny, and my daughter Tia. These individuals have stood by me through the years. My mother Bev and brother Larry are no longer with us but they will always be a part of me. Every member of my entire family is a blessing for we walked this journey together.

A thank you to my brother-in-law Jimmy for his help with the first rendition of a book cover as it represented the direction the final cover needed to take. To Rick Trelease, for his talent as a photographer in creating my author's photo. Also to my husband Dann and son- in-law Mark for improving my original logo idea for my personal author's site to create the perfect image.

Friends and members of my writing groups have my heartfelt gratitude, as their support was truly amazing. These wonderful people sat through countless revisions, offering guidance and encouragement along the way. Many even gave their valuable time and thoughts in the form of book endorsements.

Dr. Mark Doubrava and Ocularist Eric Lindsey's contribution to medical accuracy and faith in this project was invaluable.

The Next Century Publishing Team brought their expertise and dedication to my manuscript transforming it into a published book. Without them my work may well be tucked away in a drawer.

Ken Dunn (CEO) saw a need and filled it with talented people. Tiffany Magner (General Manager) stayed in constant touch teaching, encouraging and helping me every step of the way. Simon Presland's (Editor in Chief) expertise in the editing of my book was of great value as well as his kind words. Shannon Lutz (V.P. of Marketing) and her entire team's knowledge and dedication created the platforms needed to reach my readers. Rhosabelle Ocampo (Social Media Manager) and Blake Conover (Copy Writer) helped me weave my way through this unfamiliar territory. Jason Sunder (Graphic Designer) has my overwhelming gratitude for helping to create the perfect book cover. Evan Deiro (Social Media and Website Design) and Taylor Nash (Blog Posts and Press Releases) used their individual talents to make this book a success. I'm sure there were many other staff members involved in this book's development and to them I say thank you, as well as those in the areas of printing and distribution.

When the process of publication began, I had no idea how involved it was or the incredible number of people needed to produce the final work. The Next Century Publishing Team has blessed my work and me. They will always have my unending gratitude.

Through everyone's encouragement and support the dream of making this much-needed information available has become reality!

With my sincere love and gratitude,

Cynthia L. De Boer

INTRODUCTION

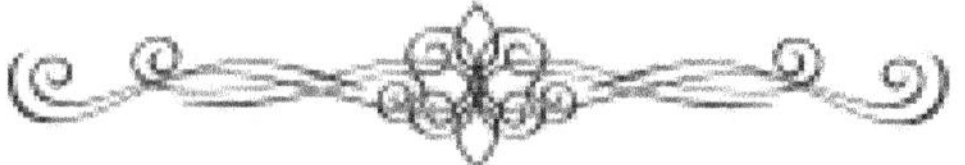

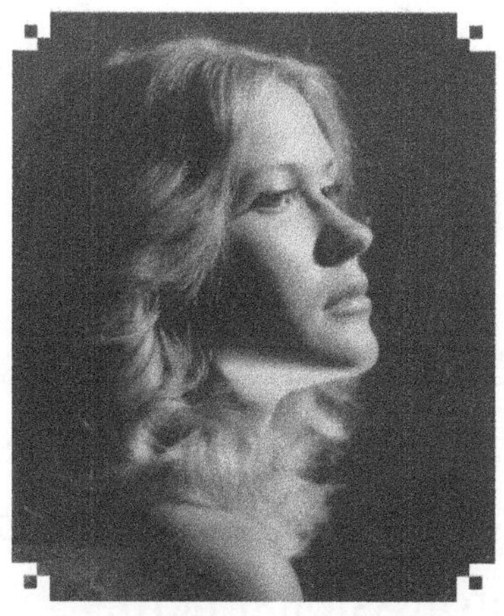

Author's photo at seventeen

after the loss of her eye

"Me, Myself and Eye" is the blending and acceptance of:

ME, the physical body...

MYSELF, the emotional mind and...

EYE, the prosthesis... into a complete and healthy being.

This is my personal journey through the fight for sight and the eventual loss of my left eye in my teens. I believe this information will be of benefit to anyone faced with this type of loss. However, please review this information before sharing it with a child, as there may be sections not appropriate for certain ages. As well, this book is *not* intended to take the place of any medical or professional help.

Information of any kind was not readily available when I lost my eye, but thankfully the Internet has become a valuable tool in understanding the medical and physical aspects of this loss. Sadly, there still isn't much written concerning the emotional and realistic sides of living with a prosthetic eye. I will address these important issues by covering the following topics:

a)   Personal perceptions of self

b)   How others may view you

c)   Instructions on care

d)   The techniques to camouflage your prosthesis

e)   How glasses can help or hinder the appearance of your eye

f)   The Phantom Phenomenons

Losing an eye is a very personal experience; which is as varied as the individuals suffering the loss. To say that this experience changes you is a given, but as I discovered at a youthful age, with the right knowledge you can adapt and allow your prosthetic eye to become a welcomed part of you and an inspiration to others.

CHAPTER 1

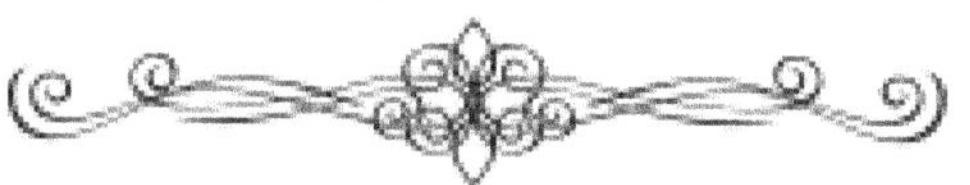

THE FITTING &

THE FIGHT

At seventeen I waited for a very special fitting. This was not for a formal dress to wear to a high school prom, but for an eye. I pretended it was an ordinary thing, something one does every day. Secretly, I was terrified!

The reality that I may lose the minimal vision in my left eye was always lurking in my sub-conscience, but the unthinkable had transpired, I lost my eye. This life-long battle for sight was over---ending in complete defeat.

According to my parents, three months after my birth in 1960 it became apparent that something was wrong with my sight. My blue eyes were growing larger and were extremely sensitive to light. A disease called glaucoma was found to be the culprit. This condition is rarely found in infants as it generally develops much later in life. Glaucoma occurs when intraocular pressure builds up in the eye, causing it to enlarge and putting pressure on the optic nerve. This results in light sensitivity, a loss of peripheral vision and blindness if not treated.

In my case, surgery was the only option. A successful surgery was performed on my right eye at three months of age and then attempted at four months on my left eye. Unfortunately, due to cardiac arrest, the surgery had to be postponed until I was six months old. By that time the pressure had increased the size of my left eye and the ticking of the clock robbed that eye of most of its sight. The optic nerve was permanently damaged. My limited sight allowed me to see the number of fingers a person would display at a distance of less than twelve inches. I was legally blind in my left eye and nothing could change that. Still my lack of sight never presented a problem, as I didn't miss what I never remembered having. Apparently, the younger you are the easier these types of transitions seem.

Glaucoma also left my right eye severely near-sighted so eyeglasses were prescribed as soon as possible. This corrected the vision in my right eye to 20/20 but nothing could be done for my left one. Since no prescription would help, a balanced lens was placed in the left side of my glasses. The balanced lens was about half the strength of the right one, making it thinner and lighter. It also helped the appearance of the glasses, while maintaining a sense of balance between the thicknesses of the individual lens. The right lens measured nearly three quarters of an inch thick, so weight was a genuine concern.

Even with nose pads, the weight of my glasses caused them to slide down my slender bridge onto my cheeks. Constant adjusting became a way of life and I can't ever remember not wearing glasses. They were just a part of me.

Daily eye drops kept my glaucoma in check until 1972. That's when another corneal decompensation attacked my weakened left eye. Corneal blisters erupted three to five times a week upon waking. You could actually see a bubble on the front of my eye before it would pop, leaving behind a concaved indentation and a great deal of pain. As my eyelid crossed over the surface of the open blister, it felt like rubbing a raw blister on your skin. Even with my eye completely closed, the slightest eye movement triggered a cascade of water and pain. These blisters remained for several hours as the cornea's healing process occurred. The blisters were consuming my entire life. I dreaded going to sleep at night not knowing what I would wake to. Was it going to be a normal day or another trip to Dr. Hix, as my excruciatingly painful eye flooded my face with tears? It seemed I was in an endless nightmare.

Dr. Ivan E. Hix M.D. had cared for my eyes from infancy and I trusted him completely. He was truly a wonderfully gifted and determined man. After researching and trying every treatment he could think of, he arranged for me to attend something called "The Rounds" at St. Anthony's Hospital in Denver. A team of doctors, all experts in their specialized fields would examine a patient, and then confer on likely solutions to the problem.

My appointment was scheduled and

the blisters erupted right on time. I sat in the darkened examining room staring into the bright lights of each physician, my eye was tearing uncontrollably and the intense light seemed to be scorching the surface of my raw eye. Doctor after doctor came and went and my pain continued. Some doctors were very sympathetic while others seemed to be looking at me like their latest science project.

Hours later, The Rounds yielded three possibilities, all of which seemed archaic. The first suggestion was to wear a wooden spool from thread around my chest when I slept.

The spool would prevent me from rolling onto my stomach, as some doctors believed gravity might be the cause. There was no change. The second idea to use a hair dryer set on low to dry out the blisters. This technique caused unbelievable pain and only made matters worse. The third and final thought was a frightening procedure, an injection of alcohol into the eye. This procedure was to be done at St. Anthony's and I will never forget the horror of seeing what appeared to be a needle the length of a sword coming at my left eye. I was told to hold completely still as any movement might cause permanent damage. It was cold and clinical. Lying there felt like I was just a specimen for yet another science project. I was scared out of my mind and my only thought was to run. The frightening procedure ended and the blisters kept coming. My hope dwindled with the last possible solution a failure.

Thankfully, Dr. Hix persisted and came up with the idea for me to continuously wear a soft contact over the affected eye. The only purpose of the contact was to serve as a bandage of sorts...and it worked! If the blisters reoccurred they were unknown to me, and life became ordinary. Truly I was grateful to Dr. Hix; his knowledge and wisdom blessed my life. It would be impossible to repay such gifts.

Several years later, this mysterious condition was identified as Fuch's Dystrophy, which affected the cornea in two ways. The first is the corneal blisters I experienced, but due to my nearly non-existent sight I'm not sure if I experienced the second, the breakdown of the cornea's endothelial cells. This results in a thickening of the cornea and doesn't allow water to naturally escape the eye. The resulting cloudy vision is like looking across a steam room. Vision is dependent on how much fluid is trapped in the thickened cornea. The more water, the more steam, the less you see. The disease can be aided with specialty drops, but eventually leads to blindness. Currently, a corneal transplant is the final option and comes with its own set of risks.

CHAPTER 2

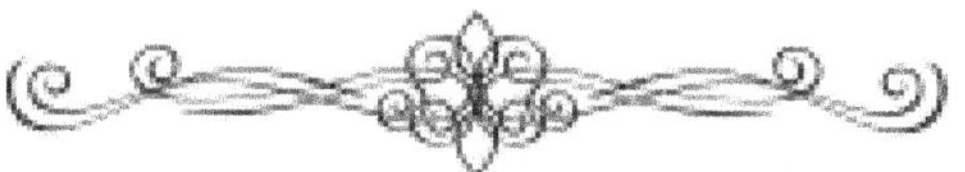

A NEW ME

During my sixteenth year a soft contact became available for my right eye. How exciting—I was on top of the world! NO MORE GLASSES!

For as long as I could remember kids teased me. The same stupid jokes were repeated over and over, but each time the person speaking acted as if they were the cleverest person in the world. Surely no one else had thought up his or her line. "Four Eyes," "Coke Bottle Girl," "I didn't know they made glasses THAT thick!" and "Can you see planets with those?" followed me everywhere. Consequently, friends were few. Writing became my solace, my escape from harm. With a few strokes of my pen, anything became possible!

I anxiously waited to see how my world would be without glasses and was truly astonished! This simple contact lens transformed me from a seemingly shy clumsy caterpillar to a bright butterfly bursting from my cocoon with excitement for my new world. The rude remarks ended. Now that my heavy glasses no longer concealed the fact that my left eye didn't track well due to its minimal sight, I did occasionally hear a lazy eye comment. Still, that was so much better!

My confidence as a young woman grew and I felt good about myself. Many of my classmates didn't even recognize me and treated me quite differently. Even some of the people who previously spouted their idiotic jokes wanted to be my friend. How can a set of thick glasses make so much difference to others? I was still the same person.

I remained close to my *pre-contact* friends and shut out the false ones. It felt great to be the one deciding, instead of being ignored because of something I wore on my face.

The contact lens not only improved my view of the physical world, but it also gave me insight into a person's character. Everything became clearer. What a wonderful gift. The world seemed right. Unfortunately, that was short lived.

CHAPTER 3

THE FINAL BLOW

Age seventeen brought with it an unexpected horror. All of a sudden, I couldn't see a thing out of my left eye and it ached. My green iris now looked a purplish color and the eye felt soft to the touch. At a very young age I learned to tell when my eye pressure raised just by pressing on the top of my closed eyelids. The firmer the eye felt, the higher the pressure, like a water balloon holding too much water. What I felt in my left eye was anything but normal; the pressure seemed non-existent.

Dr. Hix took one look and sent me to a retinal specialist. The retina is a thin layer of tissue covering the back of the eye. It's light sensitive, and if the retina has a tiny tear or a small area of detachment from its underlying layer of supporting tissue, it can be localized and repaired. This is considered a medical emergency because if treatment isn't rapid (within 24 to 72 hours), the entire retina may detach, causing blindness. Due to my minimal vision I didn't realize a problem existed. The retina had detached completely and my eye was filling with blood making the iris change color.

Back then, I didn't know anything about a retina much less what it could mean. I assumed this problem could be controlled, if not solved, with a simple procedure. Intense shock hit when I discovered it meant losing my eye. Frankly, I couldn't deal with it, so I joked about having one of Elizabeth Taylor's lavender eyes. I knew how absurd it sounded, but I would rather think of myself as a young woman with amazing eyes and not a scared teenager facing an unthinkable reality.

It seemed such a cruel joke God had played on me. All my tears, pain and time ... for WHAT? I had less than a year as a typical girl only to have it ripped away without warning. A blow to the head caused the retinal detachment, costing me my complete loss of vision and the ensuing removal of my left eye. Surgery and a glass eye—how horrific!

CHAPTER 4

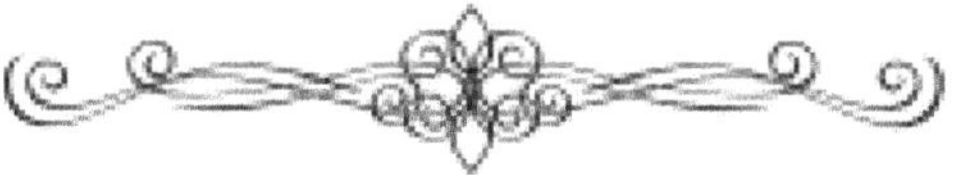

IT'S NOT JUST AN EYE

No matter how I tried to convince myself, my left eye was only a part of me and a troubled part at that. It seemed surreal. I knew no one with a glass eye. Celebrities such as Sammy Davis Jr. and Peter Falk weren't exactly poster boys for the concealment of this condition. The series *The Six Million Dollar Man* starring Lee Majors ran through my head as well. His character had a bionic eye among other body parts. Part man, part machine. Is that what I was facing? Eye patched pirates and these movie stars invaded my nightmares, and literally every moment of my day. The trauma never ended!

All the years trying to save my eye seemed so useless, and all the pain I endured was for nothing. A chance for a normal life, only to have my wings clipped so soon. Vanity came calling, and I worried how I would look and how a glass eye worked. Eyes are said to be the windows to our souls and now one of mine was going to be fake, the curtain drawn on half of my face. How would others treat me if they found out? Would my glass eye be hideously apparent? How does the eye stay in place? How does it move? How do you care for it? Does it come out easily? Am I going to have to worry about losing it if I bend over? Nothing but questions, horrible names and one-eyed jokes engulfed my mind. Why was this happening? Hadn't I sacrificed enough for my sight?

I felt God had betrayed me. My world was unfair and cruel. Family and friends were devastated by the news. The sad looks when they thought I didn't see, the hushed conversations when I entered the room and the fake smiles and laughter trying to make everything happy. It was a loss, certainly not as severe as a death, yet even though I knew nothing of the seven stages of grief, my family and I went through them.

For me the *Shock* was terrifying. The first few days blurred together as I moved through the hours on automatic pilot. *Denial* was right there too. This just could NOT be happening. There must be another solution. *Bargaining* came next, although I didn't know what to offer, as nothing seemed to hold enough value to justify the price of an eye. *Guilt* also reared its ugly head. Certainly I'd done something to deserve this, but what? What did I do to deserve this? *Anger* was a constant companion, stepping in at various degrees. For God's sake hadn't I paid for that eye with enough days of pain? It ruled my life and impacted my family's lives for so damn many days. It just wasn't fair! That's when *Depression* darkened my days and nothing brought a smile. I desperately wanted to stay in bed, after all nothing ever works out. My calculations revealed each day of happiness costs three days of suffering in my world.

I wove my way through the mix of emotions, not knowing when they would come, how long they would stay or even if they would attack in numbers spinning my head around until I was sick to my stomach. All the while I did my best to hide my emotions from those who cared for me. Adding to their grief was not an option. The final stage of *Acceptance* came slowly, but it did come, and it came as my fears of the unknown were lifted through knowledge. Some knowledge came to light over the period of several years.

CHAPTER 5

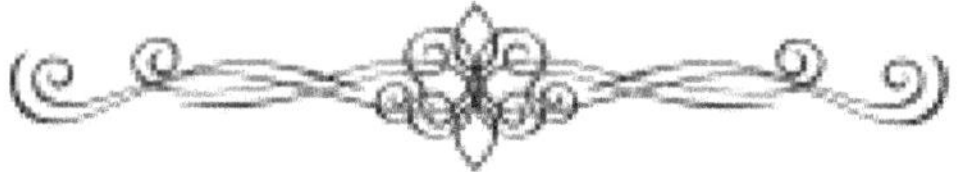

A SURGICAL GOODBYE

Late in the evening, I sat alone in a steel railed hospital bed. No position brought me comfort. Head up, head down, knees up, knees down, nothing helped. Anger filled my every cell! A 7:00 am surgery was scheduled to take out my eye. There was nothing right about this situation. The horrific thoughts taking control of my mind surely weren't helping me, so I began flipping through the TV channels and came across a re-run of a "Love Boat" episode. The lovely Sandy Duncan was starring in the show. Someone told me her left eye was glass so I watched her every movement with intensity. She had big, beautiful eyes the color of a brilliant sky. The only thing my deep observation spotted was that her left eye did not track as well as her right. A difference in tracking from one eye to the other wasn't new to me. That, I could handle. Faith instantly replaced fear. My body calmed, optimism filled my heart, and sleep came as I held her image in my mind.

The next morning is quite a blank. That's a defense I learned as a little girl. Block out the negative because you certainly cannot change it. Medical problems plagued my existence from birth, and I always believed they were an enormous source of heartache for anyone who cared for me. Pretending I was fine also became another defense and the solution to maintaining other people's happiness.

I can, however, share the details of my surgery. The optic nerve was cut, my eye removed, and a ball-shaped ocular implant was permanently embedded deep in the eye socket. The implant was held in place by surgically attaching it to the remaining muscles of the eye. After healing, a prosthetic eye would be fitted over the implant thus enabling it to move. My tear ducts were not affected and continued to function normally, allowing this natural water to maintain a moist eye socket and prosthesis.

I woke from the surgery with my eye heavily patched. The nurse told me everything went well and Dr. Hix would be in to check on me. Once again, I began acting as carefree as possible and turned my attention to the beautiful plant I brought to the hospital as a present for him. Dr. Hix tried everything to save my eye and I knew my loss was upsetting to him. I wanted him to know how much I appreciated everything he did for me. He smiled from ear to ear, saying it was the first time a patient gave him a gift for performing any type of surgery, much less the taking of an eye. I would have given him the world if I could. He never gave up on me!

After being released from the hospital, the ocular implant and eye socket needed time to heal before I could be fitted with an eye. Days seemed to run on a forty-eight hour cycle during this recovery period. However, I quickly grew sick of the sticky tape that held the metal patch, filled with holes, and the underlying gauze tightly in place. Every application of new tape ripped away another layer of my skin, leaving it incredibly raw. The tape tugged at my face with even the slightest facial movement.

I felt like a robotic human with a mechanical looking holey metal patch hiding what surely must be a blood-red socket with electric wires sparking out in all directions, waiting for a bionic orb to be attached in place of my nat- ural eye. These strange thoughts haunted my seventeen-year-old mind. I didn't want any- one to see my empty socket and certainly never wanted to look at it myself. But there was no hiding that ugly silver patch, which seemed to invite inquiries from complete strangers. My standard reply was that my eye was infected and covered to allow it to heal. Not exactly a lie, but I couldn't share my secret! Trips away from home were avoided, as I hated being questioned. All the while I wondered what lay beneath that awful patch!

CHAPTER 6

BLUE EYES & THE FITTING

The fitting for my prosthetic eye took place at Denver Optic. I sat with my mother, trying to act happy-go-lucky in the small, nondescript waiting room occupied by one other person. Machines sounding like car buffers whirled in the next room while the smell of plastics filled my nose.

My picture of the perfect man, other than Tom Selleck, was tall with a framer's muscular body and an architect's intelligent mind. To my horror, my perfect guy was the other person in the room. He stood easily six-three, in his late twenties, wearing a short sleeve plaid shirt, jeans and work boots. His wavy dark mahogany hair danced about his bright sea blue eyes, while his deep tan helped to illuminate them even more. He was simply gorgeous and I was positive he wasn't there for himself. What luck—Robot Woman meets Mr. Perfect, a scene straight from "The Twilight Zone." I prayed to be invisible or perhaps just melt into the magazine I pretended to read.

Just then a man in a white lab coat came from the back and handed Mr. Perfect a receipt saying he'd see him in three months. I nearly fell off my chair. Mr. Perfect, a patient? With those eyes? He turned looking directly at me, smiled beautifully and winked as he walked out the door. Wow! Maybe, everything would be all right.

CHAPTER 7

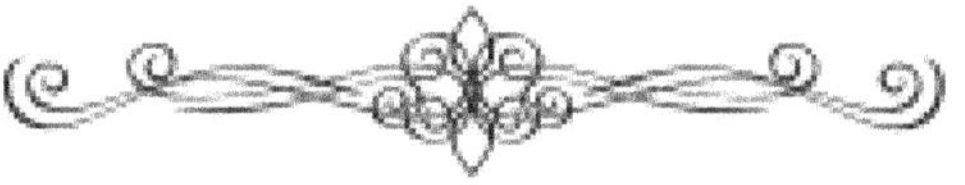

ARTISTRY AT ITS BEST

The ocular artist or ocularist, whom I will call Ted, was a middle-aged man with a kind face. He escorted me to a small table and we took seats directly across from one another. Ted went over my records, removed my patch and examined the eye socket and the movement of the ocular implant. Satisfied with his findings, he explained the process and the fact that glass eyes aren't really glass. Although they have the appearance of glass, they are a plastic composite, an acrylic of sorts. They are also referred to as an artificial eye and of course a prosthesis or a prosthetic eye. The procedure began by injecting a white substance the consistency of thick pudding into the socket with instructions to look straight ahead while holding completely still. A slender tube was placed in the thick liquid to serve as a handle for easy removal once it cured into a hard solid. The hardened substance formed the mold for the back of the prosthetic eye, creating a perfect match to the socket's ocular implant. The prosthetic eye was placed over the implant to ensure a great fit, critical for movement. Curing time took only a few minutes and made the socket feel very dry, but passed quickly.

The contour of my right eye, its shade of white, and the size and number of blood vessels were all analyzed. Next, he held up what appeared to be metal washers until a perfect match was located. The washer needed to correspond to my right eye's pupil and iris sizes exactly. Ted carefully painted the washer with tiny brushes, each with a different numbers of bristles, until it mirrored my right eye flawlessly. Ted was a true artist and I complimented him on his wonderful talent. What an amazing process. It was really quite something.

The session ended with my eye patched after a temporary clear orb was placed in the socket. The orb allowed the socket to become accustomed to having something in it.

An appointment was set to pick up the finished product and, to my surprise, I found myself feeling excited about the prospect.

The date arrived with my nervous excitement. Ted removed the patch and the clear orb, enabling him to examine the socket once more. Everything appeared to be fine, so he presented the eye created especially for me. Ted placed it into my socket and instructed me to look in several directions as he checked the curvature and movement. A few slight alterations were needed, so the eye was removed.

As I waited for Ted to return, I gathered my courage, picked up the hand mirror to examine my empty socket for the first time. Emotionally it wasn't an easy thing to see a vacant hole where part of me use to be, knowing this was reality. I blinked back the water that pooled in the corners of my eyes, wiped my face and tried to be clinical in my thinking. The best way to describe my empty socket is that it resembles a gum line after a tooth is removed. It's a concaved area of red flesh. It's as simple as that.

Within minutes Ted returned and placed my new eye back into its socket and we repeated the movement process. Pleased with the outcome this time he handed me a mirror. Water drops filled my eyes once again, but this time happiness brought them. How truly impressive! My prosthesis actually looked better than the eye I lost, as my natural eye was always a bit larger than my right eye.

Ted explained that the ocular implant aids the movement of the prosthetic eye and that the eyelid and socket are what hold it in place. Occasionally, it would need to be polished, as proteins build up on the front causing discomfort and prevents the eyelid from closing properly. A follow-up appointment would be in three months, and I should call if any problems arose before then. No other information was given. That was it, I thought. Nothing else to learn. Life would be as always. How wrong I was!

CHAPTER 8

FELINE FOCUS

Because I wore a contact, my eye movements weren't masked behind a pair of glasses. A movement too far in any direction was a dead give-away so I searched for a solution to hide this problem.

Cats revealed the key. Their eyes stay fairly fixed; it's their head that moves. Right, left, up and down. As I practiced their movements in front of a mirror, I discovered by blinking the moves became flawless as I turned my head. No one seemed to notice these subtle changes and my secret remained my own. These surprisingly simple moves worked like magic!

CHAPTER 9

EYE GLASSES - HELP OR HINDRANCE

When you are near-sighted, prescription lens make your eyes appear small. The more near-sighted, the stronger the lens, and the smaller your eyes seem.

Earlier, I stated that optometrists, trying to be kind, put a balanced lens in the left side of my glasses. The balanced lens was thinner and consequently my glasses were lighter in weight. However, the down side is that the different prescription strengths made my eyes appear to be different sizes. This is not helpful when trying to avoid negative attention. If you wear glasses, make sure both lens are identical in prescription strength. After all, your prosthesis doesn't care!

CHAPTER 10

PHANTOM PHENOMENONS

Not long after the removal of my eye, I was enjoying a wonderful day of shopping when all of a sudden someone stabbed me in the eye—or so I thought. Grabbing for my eye, I turned sharply to see my attacker. No one was there and my prosthetic eye was fine. What just happened? Instantly, panic struck. Luckily no one noticed my actions and I continued on as usual, never mentioning this strange event to anyone.

These bizarre episodes continued to happen without warning, and the stabbing pain would last from a few moments to several hours. Each time I prayed it would be the last, and each time the seemingly senseless pain became harder to ignore. I was caught up in my own horror movie, which I imagined would be titled The *Lost Eye Returns With A Vengeance.* Medical issues and now what? Was I losing my mind, too? Pride, fear and the need to protect the happiness of others kept my lips sealed.

Over a decade later I met Richard. He was a in a wheelchair. Both legs were missing, one removed half way between the knee and the hip and the other much closer to the hip.

A terrible train accident one cold rainy night nearly cost this young father his life. Richard and I became friends, and during one of our talks we commiserated on our body part losses. He explained that prosthetic legs didn't work well for him as they made his stumps sore and raw, but that "phantom pain" was something he couldn't get a grip on. His description of this illusive pain mirrored my experiences. An overwhelming flood poured down my face, releasing years of anxiety and confusion. This one conversation confirmed these incidents were normal. That day a thousand pounds of self-doubt washed away. I wasn't losing my mind.

The word "phantom" means an unreal sensation or illusion. Phantom pain is the very real feeling of pain in a limb or part of the body you no longer physically have. For most, the occurrences diminish with the passage of time. Nevertheless, the ability to deal with these dreadful attacks is difficult, since they come without warning and can literally steal your very breath.

Another phantom I have experienced is "phantom sight," or flashes of sight on my blind side. It's a split second of perfect sight where there is none. These unforeseen bursts of vision fill in the scene perfectly and occur sporadically; sometimes happening a few times a month and then not for several months at all. I've never gotten use to these magical bursts of sight, as they are startling, like someone sneaking up on you. To date, I haven't found any research on this particular condition and it is not to be confused with "phantom vision," which occurs when a person with a partial or complete loss of vision see things that aren't really there. This condition can be horribly frightening. Thankfully, in my case, my mind just completes what *is* there. These phantom phenomenons are our minds playing tricks on us. No matter how alarming they are, I will forever be amazed at the power of the human mind!

CHAPTER 11

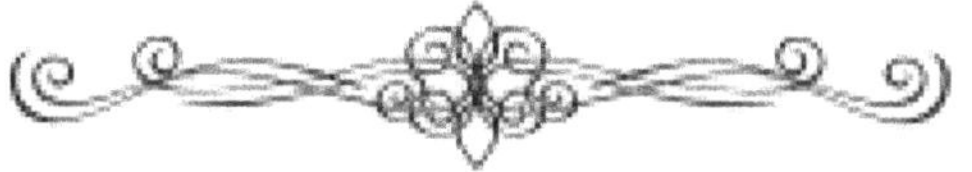

MORE TO KNOW

Most often, your eyelid will not stay completely closed over your prosthetic eye when you sleep. To date, I haven't found a solution for this but there is a lubricant available through your ocularist. The lubricant will help with eye dryness resulting from an open lid.

The emotional side for me meant that I would not allow others to see me sleeping. It's such a personal thing, so I do everything possible to shield my eye when I'm a guest at someone's home.

Prosthetic eyes are made of a very specialized plastic, but they are *not* mechanized. Consequently, they do not dilate or get bloodshot like a natural eye. When changes occur with your natural eye, your artificial eye will stay the same, so you may want to prepare for these times. Saying you have an eye infection is a reasonable response and usually ends the inquiry. Of course, if it is someone you want to share your story with, this may be a perfect opportunity to surprise him or her with your news.

Caring for a prosthesis in my case is fairly easy. In the morning or after waking I may need to wipe over the front and corners of my glass eye with a soft warm washcloth to clear out any matter or protein buildup formed during sleep.

Polishing a prosthetic eye is a needed procedure and this timeframe varies from patient to patient. Mine is done about twice a year. A polishing appointment takes approximately fifteen minutes while you wait. Polishing clears away the proteins that naturally build up on the front of the eye. Protein build up can cause the eyelid to hang up, preventing it from closing easily and is uncomfortable. If this is not addressed, the eye socket can matter and become infected. Prescription drops will then be needed to heal the socket.

Removal of a prosthetic eye is fairly easy. Your doctor or ocularist can teach you the proper placement of your fingers and what direction to look for removal. Another removal technique is to use a small suction device. This is my method of choice because of its ease in use. My eye is only removed for polishing; others may have different requirements depending on their individual medical conditions.

The aging process changes your body, including your eye socket. At seventeen, I received my first eye and I am now in my fifties. I've had a total of four eyes throughout the years. Prosthetic eyes can be solid or shell shaped. Mine is solid and works great for me. The shell type (scleral shea prosthesis) is well suited for people who have a nonworking or disfigured eye. In these cases, the shell simply covers the existing eye to serve as a cosmetic fix.

One ocularist felt the shell type would be right for me and produced my second eye. It was anything *but* right. The shell did not move as well as a solid eye because the rim of the shell was the only part touching the implant. A solid eye completely covers the implant, allowing it to move better. Also, the open space behind the shell allowed a large amount of matter to collect, creating an infection in the socket. The corners of my eye became sore and raw from the constant wiping. A third ocularist quickly replaced this uncomfortable shell with a solid eye, ending my physical troubles. Be sure to evaluate the credentials of your ocularist, as this person will be responsible for a unique and very special part of you.

Understand that your prosthesis is not a natural eye and, therefore, may look a bit different. Mine sits slightly deeper due to a deep superior sulcus, or deepening of the upper eyelid. This is a common occurrence post-surgical enucleation and is difficult to fix.

I have chosen a solution using cosmetics. It's fairly simple and can be used by everyone, male or female, no matter what age. First I use a green cover stick to cancel out any red areas around my eyes, followed by using a red cover stick or lipstick to hide any dark circles under my eyes. Next, I apply light coat of foundation to the entire eye. This coats the cover sticks and preps the eye for shadow. This enables the shadow to be applied smoothly and last longer. A dark brown matte eye shadow is then brushed into the crease of my natural eye to give the illusion of a deeper set eye, thereby creating a more balanced look. My eyes instantly appear to be more equally matched. It's amazing and quite easy to do with a bit of practice.

If you happen to wear makeup on a daily basis, you may want to complete your look with additional shadow and mascara. My eyes are extremely sensitive so I use hypoallergenic products. You may want to discuss the types of products best suited to you with your physician. Caution is best when applying anything to your skin, especially around your eyes. In regards to choosing your perfect colors, a visit to a qualified makeup artist may be in order. They can discuss your likes and dislikes to create a color pallet perfect for you.

Your hairstyle can also make a difference in your eye's appearance. Specifically, where you part your hair. For example, a center part or no part at all balances your face, making the tiniest of differences from one side of the face to the other even more apparent. This is why I part my hair on the side above my natural eye, drawing attention to it rather than my prosthetic eye.

If these tips aren't a good fit for you there is a surgical procedure called a Blepharoplasty or eyelid lift. This surgery removes skin and adds or removes fat from the eyelids. In most cases, this surgery would be performed only on the natural eye removing skin and fat to better match the eyelid covering the prosthesis. There are down sides to this surgery. Some of the possible medical complications include: infection, bleeding, scarring, and inability to close the eye, dry eye, abnormal eyelid position, and loss of vision. Also, unless the drooping eyelid impedes vision, making it a necessary medical surgery, it will be considered cosmetic in nature and is generally not covered by insurance, leaving you to foot the bill. I would recommend a thorough review of all of the facts before making this surgical decision.

In regards to my daily activities, I have noticed that when I look down for extended periods of time while reading or working on projects my eye socket can become a bit sore, which causes it to matter. I do avoid hobbies such as snorkeling or riding roller coasters. The added pressure from the water when snorkeling and the g-force from the speed of the coaster push my eye back against my implant, causing discomfort and mattering. I've never scuba dived so I cannot comment on this. I will say that it might be a good idea to remove your prosthetic eye before attempting a dive. Bouncing up and down or any jerking movement can also affect your eye, so be kind to yourself. Take on any new or old activity with this new part of you in mind, but for heaven's sake keep trying!

Mentally, adjusting to this loss may be a difficult for you or your loved ones. Counselors trained in this area may be of great value as they can help you express and understand your feelings. We all need help once in a while and if this can speed your recovery it's well worth it.

CHAPTER 12

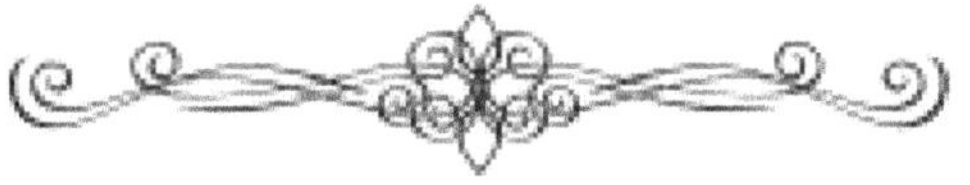

CELEBRITY STORIES

As I've stated earlier, every loss is as varied as the person experiencing it. Below are some facts about these amazing people and how they went on to fulfill their dreams. In most cases their prosthetic eyes helped their fame because people tend to remember the unusual things about someone else.

Sammy Davis Jr. was in his late twenties when he lost his eye in 1954, due to a near- fatal car accident. He made the best of it by using his eye as a source of entertainment. His humor and honesty endeared him to his fans and they remembered him because of it. How wonderfully clever!

Peter Falk's right eye had to be removed at the tender age of three. A cancerous eye tumor called retinoblastoma caused the loss. His artificial eye gave him a sexy, if not a sly look, which I loved. It also became the trademark look of his character, Columbo, and a definite asset to the role.

Lee Majors played a man with a bionic eye and thankfully, never suffered the actual loss of an eye. However, the series gave its audience hope that somewhere in the distant future we might have the ability to see without a natural eye.

Sandy Duncan does *not* have a glass eye. She did have a tumor removed from her left eye. The tumor damaged her optic nerve and caused her eye appear to be lazy or glassy. Facts I didn't learn until recently. To be quite honest, believing she did have prosthesis gave me such comfort on the night before my surgery. Sandy instantly became my inspiration, the close friend I shared a loss with and one I desperately needed that night. I don't know how I would have made it through the following days without her in my mind.

CHAPTER 13

SOME FINAL THOUGHTS

It is said that when one door closes, another opens and the loss of my eye did exactly that. In fact, the entire journey up to and after opened many doors to the unexpected. We are on this earthly journey together. Some of us may serve as fine examples of what we should strive to be, while others are the exact opposite. Both have much to teach us.

The cruel teasing I endured led me to a wonderful life of introspection and writing. Obvious changes in how others treated me, with and without glasses, gave me a genuine look into those people and their possible motives. Seeing Sandy Duncan the night before my surgery brought me comfort and hope on one of the most terrifying nights of my life. Mr. Perfect gave me a smile and the gift of assurance. Ted, the ocularist, honored me with his energy and talents by creating my perfect eye. Richard shared a very private part of himself, literally transforming my horrible thoughts into a peaceful relief. Our conversation also served as proof that fearful pride could needlessly cause years of anguish.

The dedication of so many in their individual medical fields, especially Dr. Hix, made the best of a sad situation. Dr. Hix even gave me a piece of advice once he knew I was comfortable with my new eye. He told me my new eye would come in handy when waiting for a table at a restaurant saying, "Just pop that sucker out and I guarantee you'll be seated right away!" We laughed and then he gave me a hug. Dr. Hix blessed my life!

Most importantly, my wonderful family and friend's love and support surrounded me every step of the way, comforting and enabling me to grow into the person I am today. My love for them cannot be measured for it is infinite!

Remember:

"Me, Myself & Eye" is the blending and acceptance of:

ME, the physical body---

MYSELF, the emotional mind and ---

EYE, the prosthesis, Into a complete and healthy being!

I pray this book will help you on your journey to Blend into the beautiful being I know you are!

Cynthia L. De Boer

ADDITIONAL RESOURCES

I suffered the loss of my eye in 1977 when the Internet was merely a dream of the future. Today it has grown into an expansive informational resource. When searching the web on your own, be careful to validate the authenticity of not only the site but also the information they present. Always double-check your facts.

There are a multitude of variables affecting individual patients. Due to this, each patient may want specific information relating to his or her situation. The information and resources listed below will address many common concerns.

Monetary Concerns

First and foremost, when you are gathering any type of information, my advice is to write everything down because it's easy to forget or remember incorrectly. This is especially helpful when you are dealing with an emotionally charged subject.

If insured, understanding what a particular insurance company will cover is a genuine concern. Every company is mandated by its own set of rules and benefits can vary greatly between companies. I suggest speaking with your doctor's office staff and/or ocularist first. They deal with insurance companies daily and are often your best resource for answering how a particular claim should be submitted and what benefits you may be entitled to.

After that, you may want to contact your insurance company. Armed with your new knowledge, you can now verify your benefits, get specific answers to any questions not previously thought of or answered in the past. Again, make sure you log the name of the person you spoke to, ask for a direct call back number and request written confirmation of the information you've discussed either by mail or email.

If you are not insured, the options vary due to your financial status as well as the cause of your loss. In the case of an accident when someone else was at fault, his or her insurance may step in. Victims of domestic abuse or violent crimes may receive help through the court system. But this may take some time and obviously you want to get on the road to recovery as soon as possible. I suggest exploring a victim advocacy program. These programs offer assistance with victim rights, emotional support, representation, restitution and help in filling out crime related forms as well as other resources. Check your area for these services. There are also foundations that help with funding for those in financial need. Again, you will need to do a search in your particular area.

Understanding Your Eye Disease

Many suffer the loss of an eye due to a disease. I believe understanding the disease that robbed us of our eye can ease the feelings of guilt sometimes associated with the loss. In most cases the individual did the best they could with the information available at any given moment. We simple didn't forget to lock the back door and our belongings were stolen. This is part of us and sometimes there isn't a thing we can do to prevent the loss, it just happens, due to no fault of our own. Below are some conditions that may lead to a permanent loss of vision and/or the eye itself.

Eye Tumors:

According to Eye Cancer MD. Org there are several types of tumors. Each has a specific treatment plan with many including the removal of the eye (enucleation). The following lists some tumors that may lead to eye loss: Choroidal Melanoma, Choroidal Metastasis, Melanocytoma and Iris Tumors. Another rare form of cancer is Retinoblastoma, and sadly this disease develops in children.

Retrieved from *Ocular Oncology Page* at: www.eyecancermd.org/eye_cancers.html

Fuchs' Dystrophy:

Fuchs' (fooks) dystrophy affects the cornea – the clear front window of your eye. This disorder Causes swelling in the cornea that can lead to glare, cloudy vision and eye discomfort.

Fuchs' dystrophy usually affects both

eyes and can cause your vision to gradually worsen over many years. But most people with Fuchs' dystrophy have a mid-type and don't notice much change in their eyesight.

Some medications and self-care steps may help relieve your Fuchs' dystrophy signs and symptoms. But when the disorder is advanced and you've lost vision, the only way to restore vision is with a cornea transplant surgery.

Retrieved from the *Mayo Clinic* at: www.mayoclinic.org/.../fuchs-dystrophy/ basics/.../con-2002

Glaucoma:

Glaucoma is a group of diseases that damage the eye's optic nerve and can result in vision loss and blindness. However, with early detection and treatment, you can often protect your eyes against serious vision loss.

Retrieved from *The National Eye Institute*

at:
https://nei.nih.gov/health/glaucoma/glaucom
afacts

Retinal Detachment:

A detached retina is a serious and sight- threatening event, occurring when the retina becomes separated from its underlying supportive tissue. The retina cannot function when these layers are detached. And unless the retina is reattached soon permanent vision loss may result.

Detached Retina Symptoms and Signs

If you suddenly notice spots, floaters and flashes of light, you may be experiencing the warning signs of a detached retina. Your vision might become blurry, or you might have poor vision. Another sign is seeing a shadow or a curtain descending from the top of the eye or across from the side.

These signs can occur gradually as the retina pulls away from the supportive tissue, or they may occur suddenly if the retina detaches immediately.

About one in seven people with sudden onset of flashes and floaters will have a retinal tear or detachment, according to a study reported in late 2009 in the *Journal of the American Medical Association.* Up to 50 percent of people who experience a retinal tear will have a subsequent detachment.

No pain is associated with retinal detachment. If you experience any of the signs, consult your eye doctor right away. Immediate treatment increases your odds of regaining lost vision.

What Causes Retinal Detachments?

An injury to the eye or face can cause a detached retina, as can very high levels of nearsightedness.

Extremely nearsighted people have longer eyeballs with thinner retinas that are more prone to detaching.

On rare occasions, a detached retina may occur after LASIK surgery in highly near sighted people. In a study of more the 1,500 LASIK patients, just four suffered retinal detachment; their pre-LASIK prescription ranged from -8.00 D to -27.50 D.

Cataract surgery, tumor, eye disease and systemic diseases such as diabetes and sickle cell disease may also cause retinal detachments.

New blood vessels growing under the retina – which can happen in diseases such as diabetic retinopathy – may push the retina away from its support network as well.

Sometimes fluid movement in the eye pulls the retina away.

Retrieved from *All About Vision* at: www.allaboutvision.com/conditions/ retinadetach.htm

Phantom Pain & Phantom Sight

Eye Smart obtains its information from the *American Academy of Ophthalmology*. One subject addressed is the need for doctors to reassure their patients that visions and pain are normal occurrences and not a form of mental illness. When phantom pain and sight are present it is often referred to as phantom eye syndrome. This information and much more can be found at: www.geteyesmart.org

Although the *Amputee Coalition* site is designed with the amputee in mind and refers to Phantom Limb Pain (PLP), the information on the cause and treatment of phantom pain is relevant to anyone suffering with Phantom Organ Pain (POP) from the loss of an eye. You can visit their site at: www.amputee-coalition.org

The Psychological Side of Eye Loss

When a person loses an eye, it takes a physical and psychological toil. However, far too often the psychological side of this trauma goes untreated. Patients are left with feelings of loss and grief, which they often do not understand. Such feelings are normal and visiting a grief counselor can assist the patient and his or her family. There is also an online forum that offers helpful information. You can visit that site at: www.eyeloss.com/eye- loss-grief/

More Informational Sites

The following sites contain a massive amount of information on every aspect of prosthetic eyes. I'm sure they will be of great value to you.

The American Society of Ocularists is a non- profit international educational organization founded in 1957 by professionals specializing in the fabricating and fitting of custom-made ocular prosthetics.

www.ocularist.org
1001 Mohawk St. Suite 16
Bakersfield, CA 93309
Phone: 1 (888) 973-4066
Fax: (661) 458-1660

This organization is well established and internationally recognized. They offer educational training to professionals and a publication titled the *"Journal of Ophthalmic*

Prosthetics". The web site provides valuable information to doctors, ocularists and patients. It's also a great resource when searching for a professional.

Ocularists established www.artificialeyes.net to provide support and information to people with prosthetic eyes.

This site is dedicated to patients, offering information and resources to help in adjusting to the loss of an eye. The site also contains a much-needed blog. The blog is a wonderful way to share experiences and knowledge by giving the patient a voice and an understanding that they are not alone. Patient stories are also offered through the site giving a variety of viewpoints.

Libraries

Other resources may include public, university and medical libraries. Although public libraries may be limited, they can often request specific books from other library branches. University libraries are generally accessible only to student ID holders, but you may want to contact them to request special permission to visit. Medical libraries generally provide teaching resources for medical personnel including step-by- step descriptions of medical procedures and clinical studies. The medical library I visited was located in a hospital and was open to the general public.

Word of Mouth

Finally, and I feel most importantly, there is word of mouth. You may be surprised to find that there are more people with prosthetic eyes than one might imagine. By sharing our personal stories we raise public awareness, and thereby take this often-tabooed subject out from under the dark veil of silence and bring it into the light of understanding and compassion.

In Closing

Knowledge can bring us comfort, understanding and compassion. Loss often reveals our inner strength and leads us to unexpected surprises. May your journey through this challenging time be blessed with grace, patience and love.

Blessings,

Cynthia L. De Boer

For even more information please visit

my web site and blog at:

www.cynthialdeboer.com

ABOUT THE AUTHOR

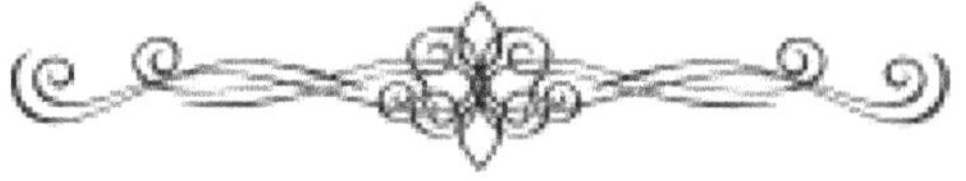

Cynthia Lee De Boer is a free-lance writer who resides in Nevada. Born in Colorado in 1960, she quickly faced numerous health challenges. These challenges as well as her varied work and life experiences have afforded her the opportunity to gain compassion and understanding of herself and others.

Writing is her lifelong passion and at times has served as an escape from the life's harsh realities. Winning an eighth grade Honor's English Medal is one of her most prized accomplishments. Cynthia continually attends conferences on the various aspects of writing. In 2011 she completed a two-year course titled "Breaking Into Print". She's also involved with writing groups and has even hosted one at a Senior Center.

Cynthia's assorted articles have been published in a local Home Magazine and one in "Shimmy", a magazine devoted to the art of belly dancing. This article journals the preparation and celebration of her fiftieth birthday where she danced for the first time in front of family and friends. She lovingly titled this inspirational piece "The Golden Dancer". It was written to pay tribute to the courage, beauty and grace of all women no matter their age.

Her story blog, (www.StoriesFromAnOpenHeart.com) was launched in 2013. The site is dedicated to short stories, fictional and non- fictional in a variety of genres. This platform gives her the opportunity to share not only her work but that of other authors as well.

Cynthia may be contacted via email at: c.deboerauthorspeaker@gmail.com